THE**FAT**TRAINER

THE FAT

HOLLAND

TRAINER

How an overweight personal trainer
finally put it all together to
get in shape.

NEWTON

Written by Holland Newton

Published by Holland Newton

For more information contact
holland@thefattrainerbook.com

First Edition April 2009 (revised December 2009)

The information in this book is true and complete to the best of
the author and publisher's knowledge. All recommendations are
made without guarantee on the part of the author or publisher.
The author and publisher disclaim any liability in connection
with the use of this information. This book is intended as a
reference to help you make informed decisions. Please consult a
qualified physician for further information.

Special thanks to the editors:
Dale and Holly Newton (newtonsbook.com)
Celeste Burnham
Ashley Henderson
Jennifer Newton

ISBN-13: 978-1-449-59198-4

This book was previously published under the same title with
the ISBN of: 978-0-557-06156-3

For Jen.
This wouldn't be possible without her.

Contents

THE FAT TRAINER

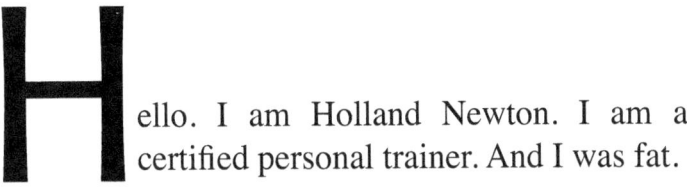

Hello. I am Holland Newton. I am a certified personal trainer. And I was fat.

This is my story. I am writing it to inspire you to live a happier and healthier life. Throughout my journey to getting in shape, I have picked up a wealth of information that can really help you and those you care about. That is my goal. After a lifetime of trying, I have finally discovered the keys to my success and I want to share them with you to help you reach your fitness goals, whatever they may be.

Holland Newton

My two-year-old son was one of the biggest motivators for me to change my lifestyle. He is also why I feel compelled to write this book, so I can share what I've learned with others who have an influence in the life of a child. Few things could be more important than helping my son establish healthy habits now as he grows and matures. I invite all parents and future parents to do what they can to give their kids the priceless gift of health and wellness. The first step in changing fitness behavior is by implementing the keys and lessons found in this book.

Holland's Tip

Get outside with your kids. Invite them to go running with you or ride bikes. Children do as they see, so let them see you being healthy. It will encourage them to be more active and also provide great bonding time.

I'm not the editor of a health magazine. I don't have a PhD, nor am I a doctor. I'm a normal person like you. I worked for three years as a personal trainer while attending the University of Missouri. I have been a very active, yet overweight individual for most of my life...until now.

How did I do it? Well, it certainly wasn't a quick fix and it definitely wasn't easy. I had to work long and hard to get this far. About a year ago, I weighed in at my heaviest weight ever. I was 26 years old and weighed more than 280 pounds! Yuck! At the time this book was published, I was a muscular 220 pounds. That means I lost 13 percent body fat. I also went from a 42" waist to a 32-34" waist. While I have not reached my weight and body fat goals, I'm almost there.

How is this book different from all of the other books out there? It might not be. But the advantage that I have is that I've lived it. I've been in the trenches. I understand the feelings and emotions of being overweight and what that means in this society. And I know that change is possible for anyone that is willing to put in the work.

This book does not, however, have all of the answers. No one does. The health and fitness industry is constantly introducing the next new thing that will "revolutionize" their industry. In just my life, I've seen the low fat, low protein and more recently, low carb trends. I have heard of berries, pills and even popcorn diets. Many of these diets work, but they typically only work short-term and can also cause all kinds of negative side-effects.

I'm a big advocate of working hard. I'm getting in shape naturally and I eat a wide variety of foods. By combining old fashioned hard work with nutrition, positive thinking and goals, I've created a program that anyone can follow to reach their fitness goals.

"There are no shortcuts to anyplace worth going."
-Beverly Sills

This book will teach you about strength training, cardio training, proper nutrition, the intangibles of wellness and goal setting. It will

THE**FAT**TRAINER

also provide ideas of how to eat better and train with more creativity. I hope the keys to my success will become the keys to your success.

Come along. Let's get fitter together.

STRENGTH

For me, there's nothing quite like finishing a tough workout— my muscles shaking, my body hungry for fuel and my mind ready to relax. I've always enjoyed strength training. It has been a great release of energy for me, a wonderful way to train for sports and a key part of the success I found as I've finally gotten into shape.

Whether you know all about lifting weights or you've never picked up a dumbbell, this chapter can give you the keys and hints to make your strength training sessions successful and to ultimately help you reach your fitness destination.

Strength

The first thing to look at when starting a lifting routine are the end goals. We must know what we want at the end in order to structure what we do in the beginning.

When I worked with clients, we always sat down to discuss their health history and set short- and long-term goals. Many people didn't really know what their goals were, so this was always a useful tool for both of us. I would then customize a program to help them obtain the results they desired.

Following are four common reasons to strength train in order to reach *your* goals.

1. Fat Loss

If you want to lose fat, you *have* to lift. Strength training burns calories regardless of your age or gender. That's what we need, right? (Nod your head.) Some studies suggest that an extra pound of lean muscle can burn as much as 50 calories per day - just to sustain itself. So, add 5 pounds of muscle to your frame and you could be automatically burning 250 extra calories every day, even when sitting or sleeping! That's a lot.

THE**FAT**TRAINER

Ask The Trainer

Why do I feel a burning sensation when I lift?

When lifting at less than 15 reps per set, the body is performing in an anaerobic state. This means that the cells of the muscle are not using oxygen to create ATP (adenosine triphosphate), but are generally using carbohydrates to create this vital muscle fuel. The byproduct of this chemical reaction is something called "lactic acid", which can be felt in the burning sensation typically associated with weight lifting.

As you build muscle mass, your scale weight will either stay the same or decrease because your body is now burning excess fat and using

Strength

it as fuel to build muscle. This is a reciprocating process. As you gain more muscle, you also gain the capacity to burn more calories, meaning you will lose more fat and scale weight.

I like to think of it like this: fat is nothingness. It just sits there. Muscle is very much alive. It needs fuel to continue to be. So while fat is sitting there mocking your self-esteem, muscle is behind the scenes trying to make you happier, healthier and live longer.

Building muscle provides a two-pronged punch in burning calories. For one, you'll burn calories while exercising and two, you'll burn calories after finishing your workout. This is because your muscles are still repairing themselves from your strength training session. During weight lifting, the muscles obtain many micro-tears, essentially breaking down the muscle. During the recovery period, which can last up to two days, those muscles need amino acids (found in protein) to repair and strengthen themselves.

THE**FAT**TRAINER

2. Slow Down the Aging Process

Face it, you're getting older. The fact of the matter is that as we age, if we do nothing to counteract nature, our bodies start to break down. Over time our bone density will begin to wane. This is one issue that can be reversed by using weight training. In order to keep our skeleton strong, we need to perform weight bearing activities such as strength training.

Holland's Tip

When lifting anything from below your waist, especially heavy things, use good posture. Lift with your legs, not your back.

3. Look Better

Like it or not, our culture puts high value in looking good and being well toned. This cultural importance weighs heavily on our own self image.

Strength

When we're confident about our own body's physical appearance, we walk a little taller, we talk a little more powerfully and we typically perform our day-to-day tasks better. Plus, when we get a chance to look in the mirror when no one is looking, we can practice our body builder poses. Strength training is one of the best and easiest ways to achieve a toned body.

4. Wellness

I'll go into this in more depth later, but strength training is only one key component of fitness. By combining lifting with a well-rounded routine of healthy living, we can achieve a wellness that can help us overcome many of life's challenges.

Holland's Tip

Work on your posture. When you're in your car, set your rear-view mirror at the angle where you're at good posture. When you notice your mirror is misaligned, adjust your posture instead of your mirror.

THE**FAT**TRAINER

Now that we have covered some of the reasons to strength train, let's get into the nuts and bolts of how to get started on a solid strength training regimen.

First, let's get some things straight. The body can be divvied up into five main muscle groups:

1. Chest
2. Shoulders
3. Back
4. Core (Abs/Lumbar)
5. Legs

More specifically, the body can be divided into these nine groups:

1. Chest
2. Shoulders
3. Back
4. Biceps/Triceps
5. Core (Abs/Lumbar)
6. Hamstrings
7. Quadriceps
8. Calves
9. Gluteus

Strength

It is important to strengthen each group for overall muscle development and health.

Ask The Trainer

Can I do crunches every day?

No - abdominals are like any other muscle. You must give them at least a day's rest in between exercises.

Lifting

Your body is an amazing interlocking and interworking network of muscles, tendons, ligaments, organs, etc. In order to stand, walk, sit-up and basically move, our muscles are busy flexing and relaxing all at the same time. When one muscle flexes, there typically is another muscle relaxing to allow the movement to occur. For example, when we flex our biceps to show off our "guns," our biceps muscle is performing a concentric contraction (flex) while the triceps muscle is elongating in an eccentric contraction (relaxation).

Depending on your age, background and abilities, lifting each muscle group 2 times per week should be sufficient. If you're a former athlete, really enjoy lifting or just want to - lift each muscle group 3 times per week.

> *"Even if you are on the right track, you will get run over if you just sit there."*
>
> *-Will Rogers*

Many of my clients were quite concerned about doing strength training in order to lose weight. The common concern I heard was that if you lift weights, you're going to get "huge." This is simply not true, especially for females. Testosterone is the muscle building buddy of body builders. Women have such a small amount of natural testosterone that in order to look like a body builder, they would have to do serious lifting, putting in hours and hours per week. They would also need serious protein supplementation

Strength

and sadly, sometimes hormone manipulation. Lifting less than three hours per week is not going to get you "ripped."

It's also useful to remember that there are basically two movements that lifting falls into: push and pull.

Pushing exercises are when you're moving the weight away from your body; pulling is moving the weight toward your body. Bench press is a push exercise. A pull-up is a pull exercise.

Holland's Tip

When grapsing a dumbbell, do not center your hand on the bar. Instead, move your hand to the outside of the weight so that the little finger is nearly touching it. This will create a more natural position and better distribute the weight.

THE**FAT**TRAINER

Balance

These factors are important to keep in mind as we build a workout routine. We always want to work balance into our routines. You may have seen a guy in the gym that is only interested in getting a chiseled chest and huge biceps. He will work these muscles over and over and he will see results. But by not working the other side (the mid-back and triceps in this case), the lifter is creating a physiological imbalance. Not only will he start to hunch over because his muscles are so big on the front side of his body, but he'll also be much more prone to injury.

So, remember, while it's nice to work out your favorite muscles, don't neglect the companion muscle, which is typically located on the opposite side of the body.

Form

There are times I just cringe when I'm at the gym because some folks have such poor form. I give them credit that they're there, but they're wasting so much of their time and putting

Strength

themselves at risk of injury by lifting with incorrect form.

While each piece of equipment has its own adjustments, there are some hard and fast rules that apply to most movements.

> #1 Be tall. Keep your shoulders down and back. "Align your spine" means to adjust your neck so your head is over your shoulders and not jarring out over your chest. Keep your chin up and look straight ahead.

> #2 When standing, keep your feet about shoulder width apart, point your toes and go easy on the knees, meaning, DON'T LOCK YOUR KNEES!

> #3 Relax. Don't tense up your muscles.

> #4 Pull abs in. Keep your abs taut against your spine and internal organs to keep them safe and to provide a solid base from which to perform your movement.

THE**FAT**TRAINER

#5 Smile. Okay, you don't always have to smile, but at least pretend that you're enjoying yourself.

Regardless of what you're doing, try to practice good form. Computers and desks are the worst culprits, with driving close behind. Try to apply the above rules even when you're not "fitnessing."

Ask The Trainer

How can I reduce post-workout soreness?

Stretch. Take a few minutes after your workout to loosen up your tight and tired muscles. It will help prevent injury and you'll feel better the next day.

Strength

Breathing

Again, individual adaptation may warrant adjustment and there are some lifts that require alternate breathing, but overall, here is a good rule to follow: BREATHE! Sounds simple, right?

Ask The Trainer

What's an easy way to make exercise more enjoyable?

Use an iPod! Listening to your own music is a great way to distract you from those exercises you don't enjoy.

Actually, one of the most neglected parts of exercise, especially while strength training, is proper breathing. Take a few minutes every now and again to focus on how you breathe rather than the weight you're moving. Optimal breathing for most movements is exhaling on the pushing/pulling or working phase and inhaling on the relaxing stage. The better we breathe, the longer we'll be able to perform a movement. Why? As the muscle exhausts its own energy stores, it needs oxygen to continue to move. Otherwise it will fail sooner. Don't believe me? Think how long you'd last if you held your breath for an entire set of a lift.

Speed

The speed at which you perform your lifts should match the tempo of your breathing. Typically, when strength training, you want a slow and steady pace. There are some variations of when to lift at a more advanced speed.

Explosion training is typically only done by athletes. This kind of training involves getting into a set position with weights, like a clean, then rapidly pushing or pulling the weights away from gravity to develop the fast twitch muscle fibers of the athlete's body. This is intended to simulate game-time activities of explosion to dunk a basketball or drive off the line of scrimmage or dive into a pool.

Negative training is a type of training that

Strength

is meant to exhaust muscles beyond what they can do using normal repetitions. These types of movements typically require a spotter because they involve moving more weight away from gravity than can be done alone.

Now you know the basics of strength training and how I used it as one of the components to finally help me get in shape. Strength training is very useful and can actually be enjoyable if you know what you're doing. If you feel inexperienced, just get in the gym and start.

Holland's Tip

Talk often and honestly with someone you trust about your experiences and challenges. Changing years of sub-healthy choices takes a lot of time. Thinking and talking about the changes will help them sink into your psyche.

Most gyms will offer some kind of free training opportunity, whether it is a complimentary session or trial offer. If those kinds of situations ever present themselves, take 'em! Sure the trainer will probably try to sell to you, but I think it is always worth it to get a little kick in the pants and to learn some new and fresh ideas.

If you're not in a position to hire a trainer, it is also worth it to invest every 6-12 weeks in a session to help stay on track. Most reasonable training sessions are going to be $70 or less for a one time shot. (The price typically jumps way down the more sessions you commit to purchasing.)

Strength

Types of Lifts and Movements:

Compound: *Using more than one muscle group at a time.*
e.g. Squat engages nearly the entire lower body, lower back and abs.

Isolation: *Using one muscle group at a time.*
e.g. Bicep curl.

Rep: *(short for repetition) One movement away and toward gravity.*

Set: *A group of reps done without resting.*

Super-Set: *(traditional) Doing one set of an exercise, then moving directly to another set of a similar exercise without resting between sets.*
 e.g. Set of bench press (chest) reps followed directly by a set of dumbbell fly's (chest).

Super-Set: *(push-pull) Instead of working a similar muscle group two sets in a row, do a push then a pull with no rest in between.*
e.g. Set of bench press (chest) reps followed directly by a set of dumbbell rows (back).

Drop Sets: *Instead of resting between sets, "burn-out" your muscles by lowering the resistance after a series of reps.*

THE**FAT**RAINER

Circuit Sets/Training: *Circuit training is similar to push/pull supersets but with minimal rest periods in between sets. It is also common to complete a one set "circuit" of a full body workout before repeating the sets again.*

Monster-Set: *A traditional superset with a third "active rest" set.*
e.g. Set of bench press (chest) reps followed directly by a set of dumbbell fly's (chest) followed directly by crunches (abs).

Interval Training with Cardio: *Performing one or more sets and then performing a set time or distance in cardio.*
e.g. Two chest press sets followed directly by running a mile followed directly by two lat pulldown sets, etc.

Periodization: *It is useful to adjust your lifting routine about every six weeks. The body has an incredible ability to adjust and make things easier for itself. It will do this with your lifting routines, so change it up.*

Rest Days: *Always rest at least a day in between lifting muscle groups. This allows ample time for the body to work its magic to repair those damaged muscles, all while burning calories and making you stronger.*
e.g. If you do chest lifts on Monday, don't do them again until at least Wednesday.

Strength

One of the most common questions that I get is, "How long and how often should I work out?" This is a really hard question to answer in a book. Time constraints, schedules, abilities, styles, etc. are all very different with each person.

Generally speaking, try to do cardio for <u>at least</u> 180 or more minutes per week. This could be three days at one hour per day, five days at 36 minutes per day or any other combination.

As for strength training, two to three times per week is typically good. This, too, can be quite varied. For more specific suggestions for your individual needs, meet with a trainer or drop me a line at:

thefattrainerbook.com

While every person has different needs, goals and abilities, I've put together some sample routines for you to take a look at. Feel free to mix and match ideas to meet your own goals.

Visit *TheFatTrainerBook.com/routines* for more ideas and routines.

THE**FAT**TRAINER

Routine 1 - Weight Loss (Beginners)

Cardio:

Your choice. On your off days, try to choose a low intensity activity such as golf or bowling.

Strength Routine:

2 sets x 15 reps each

1. Chest Press (pecs & triceps)
2. Row (back & biceps)
3. Leg Press (entire lower body)
4. Shoulder Press (delts & triceps)
5. Lateral Pull-Down (back & biceps)
6. Stationary Lunges (entire lower body)
7. Crunches on Floor (abs)
8. Back Extension on Roman Chair (lower back)

Monday	Cardio: 30 minutes Strength: 30-45 minutes
Tuesday	Cardio: 45 minutes
Wednesday	Cardio: 30 minutes
Thursday	Off
Friday	Cardio: 30 minutes Strength: 30-45 minutes
Saturday	Cardio: 45 minutes
Sunday	Off

Strength

Routine 2 - Advanced/Power (Athlete)

Day	Lift	Reps	
Monday	Dumbbell Chest Press	12x12x10x10	
	Incline Dumbbell Press	12x12x10x10	
	Chest (Your Choice)	12x10	
Tuesday	One-Arm Dumbbell Row	12x12x10x10	
	Front Pulldown	12x12x10x10	
	Back Extension	12x10	
	Double Crunch (Stability Ball)	12x12x10x10	
Thursday	Squat	12x12x10x10	
	Leg Extension	12x12x10x10	
	Romanian Deadlift	12x12x10x10	
	Leg Curl	12x12x10x10	
	Seated Calf Raise	10x10x10	
	One-Leg Standing Calf Raise	10x10x10	
Friday	Alternating Dumbbell Curls	12x12x12	
	EZ-Bar Curls	12x12x12	
	Biceps (Your Choice)	12x12	
	Lying Triceps Extension	12x12x12	
	Triceps (Your Choice)	12x12x12	
	Bench Dip	12x12	
Saturday	Military Press	12x12x10x10	
	Upright Row	12x12x10x10	
	Bent-Over Lateral Raise	12x10	
	Crunch	12x12x12	
	Decline Sit-Up	10x10x10	

THE**FAT**TRAINER

Cardio: Your choice 30-60 minutes at least 5 times per week

	Set 1	Set 2	Set 3	Set 4

CARDIO

Unlike weight lifting, cardiovascular training has never been my strong point. It always seemed like it was such a chore. But, cardio is the reason I'm writing this book. In all of the hours and hours I spent running in the last year or so, my thoughts were filled with ideas of how I could share my story to help others dramatically improve their quality of life. I came up with the title, structure and tone of the book all while doing cardio. You can say I have a love-hate relationship with this form of training, but I'm so grateful for it and enjoy it much more than I ever did before.

Cardio

This chapter has some tips that I found very useful to help me form a better relationship with cardio training. Skipping cardio exercises will dramatically decrease your chances for success in regards to health and fitness.

Cardio is short for cardiovascular and is synonymous with aerobic training. In a nutshell, cardio training is elevating your heart rate without using weight resistance. So, running, biking, swimming, kick-boxing, aerobics and skiing are all types of cardiovascular training. Aerobic essentially means that your body is able to provide enough oxygen to your muscles for them to perform the desired function.

Cardio training is optimal for fitness because it is how we can burn calories for an extended period of time. Because the body is using oxygen

Holland's Tip
Try sprinting up hills then jogging back down. This is a great way to add variety to running.

as its fuel source, we can perform cardio exercises for 10, 30, even 60 plus minutes.

Heart Rate

The most effective way to perform cardio training is using your heart rate as a guide. The easiest way to calculate your heart rate is by following this formula:

220 - your age = your maximum heart rate

For example - I am 27 years old so ...
220-27=193. Therefore 193 beats per minute (bpm) is my maximum heart rate. There is really never any need for me to ever go higher than that.

The optimal cardio zone is between 60 percent and 85 percent of your max. Again, in my case:

$$193 \times .6 = {\sim}116$$
$$193 \times .85 = {\sim}164$$

So as I exercise, I try to maintain a pace that keeps my bpm as close to 164 as possible because

Cardio

the closer you can get to and maintain that 85 percent mark, the better. Most of my untrained clients had no problem reaching and exceeding the 85 percent threshold with minimal effort, so remember, as you start out, keep your eye on that heart rate and adjust your effort accordingly.

Prolonged levels much higher than 85 percent isn't typically advised for weight loss goals. This is because the body begins to use other sources to fuel the muscles because oxygen cannot be supplied rapidly enough to the cell. While this may sound like it's good, it actually doesn't burn as many calories as that magic 85 percent level.

Ask The Trainer

Are there other options besides working out at 85% of my max?

Yes. Try interval training. Exercise at your highest intensity for as long as you can, then "rest" at about 50-60 percent for a couple minutes. Repeat throughout your workout.

THE**FAT**TRAINER

Athletes, especially those that use sprinting activities, often train at higher heart rate levels to increase their performance at race/game time.

Just remember that while exercising at a lower heart rate is okay, for optimal calorie burn during and after a workout, shoot to be around 85 percent of your maximum heart rate.

Measuring Heart Rate

There are several ways to track your heart rate. Most cardio equipment in gyms have sensors where you can place your hands. While these are somewhat accurate, they require you to be holding the sensors while exercising, which isn't always easy and/or reasonable.

Another method is the old fashioned way. Manually checking your pulse is most easily done on the artery in the neck (called the carotid pulse). Place your forefinger and middle finger in the middle of the triangle formed by your jaw, throat and the big muscle on the side of your neck (sternocleidomastoid). Press just firmly enough to feel the pulse. With a little practice, you'll be able to find your pulse almost right away. Once

Cardio

you find your pulse, count the number of beats you feel in 15 seconds. Take that number and multiply it by four to get your beats per minute.

The third and best way to check your pulse is to invest in a heart rate monitor. These monitors consist of two pieces: a chest strap and a receiver (watch). I purchased my first monitor at Walmart a few years ago for about $60 (US) and I've seen the same model for less than $50 now. The price is well worth it!

There are few pieces of equipment that make as big of an impact on fitness training as heart rate monitors do. It takes a lot of the guess work out of working out. I found that before I purchased the monitor, I was working harder than I needed to. This meant that I got tired more quickly, I wasn't able to work out as long, I didn't burn as many calories and ultimately, I didn't lose as much fat as I wanted.

Once I was able to constantly monitor where my heart rate was, I was able to pace myself accordingly and go for longer, more effective workouts.

So, try to always be on top of your heart rate and you'll be much more prepared to reach your goals.

THE**FAT**TRAINER

Ask The Trainer

Should I work out in the fat loss zone to lose more weight?

For optimal weight-loss results, maintain a heart rate near the upper range of the cardio zone. Exercising at that intensity will burn more TOTAL calories over time than the fat loss zone.

Cardio Options

The key to cardio is not just focusing on calories (they are important of course), but finding something that you can do and at least kind of enjoy. Softball, tennis, walking, flag-football, rappelling, soccer, etc. are all good options to mix in with more intense cardio workouts during your week.

Were you a jock in high school/college? Find a rec or church league of your sport. I love playing basketball. While I'm playing, I understand that

Cardio

I'm not using the time as calorically efficient as I could with just straight running, but I love playing ball. If you're doing what you love, there is a much higher likelihood that you're going to keep doing it.

Below are my preferred options for cardio training:

1. Biking

Whether it's indoors or outdoors, mountain or road, biking is a great form of exercise. It's low impact, which means those with bad knees and hips can participate and still get a good cardio workout.

"Even if you fall flat on your face at least you are moving forward."
-Sue Luke

THE**FAT**TRAINER

2. Ellipticals

Another great low impact workout is on elliptical machines. There are dozens of different kinds, but they all follow the basic idea that your feet never leave the standing pedestal and they follow an elliptical motion.

Ask The Trainer

I prefer swimming. How should I track my heart rate?

Swimming is a great low impact exercise. For tracking heart rate, most heart rate monitors can be used in water. That's your best bet.

---

3. Stairs

I really enjoy running stairs outside in a football stadium. The problem is that there aren't a lot of empty, open and large stadiums out there.

Cardio

Stair climbers are the next best thing. So, whether you are on the real thing or a stair climber, this is a great workout.

Ask The Trainer

What's the best way to measure fitness?

While a scale is okay, VO2 max, strength, speed, etc. are all really good options, too. Body fat percentage is the best standard of measurement to go by.

---

4. Running

Now, you may cringe when I mention running, but running is one of the best ways to burn calories, especially if you're keeping your heart rate at about 85 percent of your max.

THE**FAT**TRAINER

Why Run

When I was at my heaviest, I didn't like running at all. It was hard. It was really hard. It was too easy to get out of breath and I couldn't go for very long. It just wasn't fun! I knew that it was good for me though, so I stuck with it. And guess what? I got better and it got easier. I went from running a 10 minute mile to a mile in 6 minutes and 19 seconds in a matter of a couple of months. Sure, it helped that I dropped 20 or 30 pounds, but more so, my body adjusted to running and I actually started to enjoy it.

Holland's Tip

Let go! By holding onto the cardio equipment, you minimize the efficacy of your workout by reducing how many muscles can be in action. This is especially true on stair climbers or treadmills at a high incline. Holding onto the machine is certainly fine when changing speed or resistance, but let go whenever possible. You'll get a better workout and get fitter faster.

Cardio

One thing that really worked for me was to set goals and targets each time I ran. Sometimes I wanted to beat my mile time. Other times I wanted to see how far I could run before being just too tired. Other times I would try to beat three or four miles in a certain time limit. I recorded all of these times which gave me small targets to aim at for the next time. I strongly encourage you to give running a try. Be disciplined with it for a month and you'll see results.

Holland's Tip

Don't be afraid to park further away at the store or mall. Instead of driving around looking for the closest spot, just park the car and walk. It's one way to add a little extra movement to your day.

Form

Correct form is important to learn from the get-go. Try to run with your toes pointing straight forward and try to stride evenly along your foot.

THE**FAT**TRAINER

Don't put all of your weight on the inside or outside of your feet. Your upper body posture is also important. Stand tall and relaxed with a slight forward lean. Move your arms forward and backwards instead of up and down. Avoid clenching your fists and try to be relaxed and fluid.

Shoes

Another important part of running is having the right shoes. I highly recommend going to a shop that does a video gait analysis. This is where they put you on a treadmill and film your cadence for slow-mo replay and analysis. If the shop knows what they're doing, they will then be able to recommend a handful of shoes that would be right for your running style and also suggest techniques to tighten up any miscues in your running form. You may pay a little more for these types of shoes and service, but I believe it's worth it.

Socks

Let me touch on the oft-forgotten ally to good shoes: good socks. This is one of the gems I took

Cardio

away from my time getting the gait analysis at my shoe shop. Runners and exercisers in general should wear synthetic socks. (It doesn't matter if they're thick or thin, short or long.) Cotton socks are good for wearing around the house or making puppets, but not for sweating in. When cotton gets wet, it absorbs and retains the moisture. Imagine two sponges wrapped around your feet. Doesn't sound like it'd be too easy to run, does it? NOPE! Shoes are designed to keep your feet as dry as possible. By wearing cotton socks, you're minimizing the drying functions of shoes. Plus, when cotton absorbs water, it expands and doesn't keep its shape. This is just a breeding ground for blisters and sadness.

Holland's Tip
Take the stairs instead of the elevator. This will give your heart and lungs a bit of a challenge.

THE**FAT**TRAINER

Where to Run

As to where to run, I'll leave that up to you. I prefer running on a track or out on a trail. I like treadmills the least but am resigned to use one in poor weather. Oh, and don't let people tell you that it is unhealthy to run in cold weather. It's simply not true. If you're able to layer up appropriately, your lungs and other innards are well equipped to handle low temperatures. Be careful about slippery conditions and cover any exposed skin. Try it. It's kinda fun to be out running in the crisp air.

"If you went running when you first started thinking about it, you'd be back by now."

-Nike ad

Cardio

If you're like most people, getting out the door is the hardest thing. Even when I don't want to work out, I'm *always* grateful that I did afterwords. My biggest suggestion for you? Just get out and do it. It *will* get easier.

THE**FAT**TRAINER

Holland's Tip

There are a few things to remember as we utilize the scale in our fitness routines.

1. Our body weight can fluctuate as much as two pounds in a day.

2. Try to weigh yourself at the same time of day.

3. Always use the same scale and try to stand on it the same way each time. (On the little $10 one that I have, I can lose five pounds just by changing my foot position.)

4. Keep in mind that workouts and eating times can alter what the scale says.

5. Weighing yourself too frequently can be discouraging. Many trainers recommend weighing no more than once per week.

NUTRITION

Nutrition is perhaps the most overlooked portion of fitness. We are very unaware (as a society) about what we eat. We don't know what's in it, don't know how it's made and many times don't want to know and couldn't care less. Even if we knew what was in a certain meal, we are very misinformed about whether or not it's good for you.

So, what should we eat? Good, healthy, natural foods. Pretty simple, right?

Well, not for me. I knew enough to know that there were good and bad things to eat, but I didn't know the ins and outs as to WHY we

Nutrition

should eat more of the good stuff and less of the bad. Because I didn't know the "why's," I never found the motivation to eat healthier.

The turning point for me nutritionally was a book given to me by my father-in-law. I still remember my first reaction when my wife showed me the book. I thought, "Oh dear, what new fad is it this time?" The Abs Diet by David Zinczenko proved to be far from just another fad or diet. It answered many of the "why's" behind healthy eating and helped catapult my wife and I into our new lifestyle.

Holland's Tip

Try using salad plates instead of dinner plates at everyday meals. This will help you limit your portion size.

As I read Zinczenko's book and learned more about the food I ate and when to eat it, I finally saw results that I had never seen before. I started feeling in control and enjoyed eating a wider variety of foods. It was definitely a life changing book.

In a nutshell, Zinczenko breaks down nutrition into 12 easy to remember categories called power foods:

oatmeal	*lean meat*
beans/legumes	*natural peanut butter*
almonds and other nuts	*olive oil*
leafy greens	*whole grains*
low-fat dairy	*whey*
eggs	*berries*

These power foods are nutrient dense and actually help increase the productivity of our bodies. By combining these power foods into every meal that we eat, our bodies are able to utilize the nutrients more efficiently as we work on getting more fit.

After making the decision to eat better, the first few times my wife and I went grocery shopping, it took us hours because we were trying to apply our new knowledge. We were shocked with how many preservatives and artificial ingredients were in foods that were supposed to be "good" for you.

Nutrition

It got easier with time, though and now it is pretty much second nature. We know what to look for in nutrition labels and ingredient lists, what ingredients to avoid and what is truly whole grain. We have also learned the importance of using an eating schedule and adding variety to the menu.

The next few pages explain some of the things that we've learned:

Ask The Trainer

How many calories should come from carbs?

Our bodies primarily use carbohydrates to function. About 55-65 percent of our calories should come from carbohydrates.

THE**FAT**TRAINER

Nutrition Labels and Ingredient Lists

Get to know your nutrition labels and ingredient lists. They are full of information that can really help you make informed decisions. Try these tips:

- Don't just look at the calories - compare the serving size too (typically in grams).
- Saturated fat is useful but only in small quantities, so minimize its consumption as much as possible.
- Trans fat is just bad - avoid it.
- Poly- and mono- unsaturated fats are good. These fats are found in things like almonds, fish and olive oil. They are good

Holland's Tip

Feed your kids the same things you eat. By feeding them a wide variety of healthy foods, you'll give them the priceless gift of healthy eating that they can take with them for the rest of their lives. Just make sure they are eating the right serving size for their age and size.

Nutrition

for you, but fat has 9 calories per gram, so it's very caloric.

- Look for whole grains and natural ingredients near the top of the list.
- Avoid artificial and chemical ingredients.
- Typically the shorter the ingredient list, the more natural the product.

High Fructose Corn Syrup

I don't like picking on one product, but from my own qualitative research, High Fructose Corn Syrup (HFCS) is a bad guy. Essentially, it is sugar derived from corn with a bunch of dodgy tag-alongs. This altered sweetener can be found

Ask The Trainer

How do I keep from over-eating?

Slow down and enjoy your food. By chewing it more, your body will be tricked into thinking that you are eating more than you really are.

in just about everything which makes it hard to avoid completely. Candy, soda and sweets all contain the stuff. Bread, cereal, flavored milk and crackers are all big culprits, too.

Holland's Tip

Preview what you will eat before the day and then review what you ate at the end of the day. Recommit yourself if necessary.

One of the worst things about HFCS is that it's actually sweeter than natural sugar. This is particularly bad because it dulls our sense of what is naturally sweet. So what? HFCS causes us to lose the desire for naturally sweet things, like fruit and makes us yearn for artificially sweetened things that aren't good for the body. It's very much like an addiction. There is a pretty good debate going on online about HFCS, but I avoid the sweetener and feel confident that by doing so, it has helped me lose more weight and I've been able to reign in my sweet tooth.

Nutrition

Here's another reason why reading the nutrition label will be a lifesaver. If you have to buy a product with HFCS, the further down it is on the ingredient list, the lower the amount there is in the product. An easy shortcut: there cannot be HFCS in anything that says "All Natural" or "Organic" since it "ain't natural!"

Sugar

Along with watching for HFCS, try to keep the added sugar intake to a minimum. It's impossible to cut it out completely and I don't think you should. Sugar tastes good and can help us feel good. It is also a quickly digested source of energy. When you do eat food with added sugar, try to make it as natural as possible. Remember, packages that say "All Natural" or "Organic" are your good friends.

It is important to note that when it says "sugars" on the nutrition label, it doesn't necessarily mean that sugar has been added. Fruit is full of natural sugar and that is okay. Just be mindful of the calories consumed.

Holland's Tip

Drink water. Most people need to drink more of it. I find that drinking cool water quenches my thirst better, thus allowing me to drink more of it.

Whole Grains

Another great mistake consumers make is buying things that say something like "made with whole grains" and then think that they are getting the best possible version of the product. If the first ingredient on the list isn't whole grain wheat (or oats, or corn, etc.) it is NOT 100 percent

Nutrition

whole grain. Many breads and cereals trick us into thinking that we are eating a full portion of whole grains when we really aren't.

Whole grains are good for you because:

- They are the way nature intended them to be consumed.
- They are minimally processed.
- They are typically full of nutrients, unlike processed products whose nutrients have been stripped away.
- They typically contain more fiber.
- They are tasty.

Calories

Plain and simple, the only way to lose weight naturally is by burning more calories than we consume. Sounds easy, right? Well, I guess that depends on how in-tune we are with what we eat. The easiest and most effective way to ensure that we're eating just enough to give our bodies the energy it needs to perform its day-to-day functions, as well as become a calorie-roasting machine, is by counting calories. With a little practice and awareness, this isn't really as hard as it may sound.

The difficult thing is figuring out how many calories you need to maintain your weight and body fat percentage. This is where a personal trainer can really help. There are also several reliable sites online that can estimate how many calories you need per day to stay the same weight. For complete accuracy, have your Basal Metabolic Rate (BMR) tested at your local gym or doctor's office.

Holland's Tip

Just because your bowl or plate is the size it is, it doesn't mean that it has to be filled with food. Try following the serving suggestions on the packages the food came in. The biggest culprit in my house is the cereal bowl. It is filled to the top no matter what size it is. Shrink your serving sizes (but not so low you go hungry) and you will shrink your waist.

Nutrition

Doing a search for BMR calculators online usually tends to be a good starting point. For example, a 130 pound, 5' 5", 29 year-old female needs about 1,400 calories per day to maintain her weight. To lose 1 pound per week, she'll need to have a caloric deficit of about 500 calories per day. A pound of fat is said to be about 3,500 calories. If she creates a caloric deficit of 500 calories per day, she can lose about one pound of fat per week (500 x 7 = 3,500).

Holland's Tip

The biggest portion on your plate should be veggies. They are nutrient dense and calorically low. Remember to have carbs, fats and proteins at every meal, too.

This caloric deficit can come from a combination of caloric intake reduction and added exercise or from increased exercise alone. Someone this size should not eat 500 calories less per day. One or two hundred calories may be appropriate. Ask your doctor for more advice.

THE**FAT**TRAINER

Calories Eaten - Calories Burned = Weight Gained/Lost

Eat Often

Eating often was one of the hardest things to adjust to. I had always heard that you should eat five to six small meals per day but never really understood why. Below are some of the reasons.

Ask The Trainer

What if I've got the munchies, but I'm not really hungry?

Chew on some gum or suck on hard candy. This will help keep your mouth occupied until it is actually time to eat. (Don't tell your dentist where you heard this.)

Think of your body as an old fashioned locomotive that runs on coal or wood. In order to get that big train moving, you've got to get the

Nutrition

fire hot with fuel. But in order to *keep* the train moving, you can't just give it big doses of fuel every four or five hours. You must keep the fire stoked with the fuel it needs to keep chugging along.

Holland's Tip

Believe it or not, ice cream isn't the worst thing in the world. Look for the all natural brands and then enjoy it a few spoonfuls at a time. Remember that it is the portion size that can get you into trouble, not the ice cream itself.

So it is with our bodies. First and foremost, we need to get the body going after the eight to ten hour fast we do every night. We must eat breakfast—a balance of carbs, proteins and fats. Once we get the fire of metabolism hot, we shouldn't wait four or five hours until lunch rolls around. We need a mid-morning snack to refuel the lost energy. This should consist of at least some sturdy carbs and protein. Good fats (like omega 3 and 6) are a good thing, too. Something like an apple and scoop of peanut butter covers that well.

As we perform our daily actions, we take all of these nutrients and calories and convert them into the energy we need to perform.

The way society has taught us to eat is wrong! Too many of us eat only three meals a day. Many others eat only one or two meals a day. This is just mean to your body. Over time, eating less than four meals per day trains the body to always be conserving. By restricting eating in this way, the body will take whatever nutrients it has and instead of burning them, it will store them as fat because it is worried that it won't get food again for awhile.

Act Like a Baby

This is one of the rare times when I encourage you to follow an infant's example. If you've had children, you know that they eat a lot. Newborns eat as often as every two hours. This is what is natural. It is the way they got energy and grew in the womb. They were constantly nourished. I think eating every two hours may be a little

Nutrition

excessive for a grown adult, but every three or four is more along the lines of what we're talking about.

If you're in the lucky position that my wife and I are in, don't wean your children off of the schedule of eating every three or four hours. It'll save them from all kinds of potential health issues down the road if they know how to eat instinctively.

We also need to maintain an even blood-sugar level. If we only eat breakfast, lunch and dinner, we typically will have a peak of energy soon after eating, but then an energy slump two or three hours following consumption. If we replace that energy slump with nutrients, we can maintain an even-keel of energy throughout the day and lessen the risk of diabetes.

Holland's Tip
Try eating fresh fruit and/or vegetables at every meal. Pair them with yogurt or cheese.

THE**FAT**TRAINER

Here's a good cookie-cutter schedule to follow:

7 a.m: Breakfast
10 a.m: Mid-morning snack
Noon: Lunch
3 p.m: Mid-afternoon snack
5 p.m: Dinner
7 p.m: Evening snack

At the end of the chapter, take a look at an actual week-long meal plan we use in our home.

Eat a Variety of Foods

Something that really helped me as I got used to eating six meals per day was the ability to mix it up a little. While using a schedule took the guess-work out of meals, it also gave us a reason to try new recipes and combinations. I am eating things that I never thought I would like, not just 'cause they're good for me, but because I actually like the taste.

As you get used to eating more natural, whole and organic foods, your body will adapt to

Nutrition

them and you will find that you will prefer these delicious foods over many of your past meal choices. For example, I always assumed that unsweetened applesauce would taste gross, but now, it's all we buy because the sweetened kind is too sweet.

Fuel Pre- and Post-Workout

Since working out is the time that your body is consuming the most calories, be sure that it has enough energy to perform what you're asking it to do. By having fuel in your system before you workout, you'll be more intense, have better form and be able to perform longer.

Also try to eat soon after working out. Your body is craving quick energy when a workout is finished and if you give it that energy, your body will be more efficient at burning extra calories.

As a general guideline, try to eat as soon as you can before and after exercise. This is different for every person, so take some time to get to know how your body reacts. I typically can eat a snack 15 to 30 minutes before working out and I can eat shortly after exercising.

THE**FAT**TRAINER

Holland's Tip

Vacationing or business trips can create havock on healthy living. While packing, prepare a bag full of healthy and travel friendly food.

Here are some foods we like to pack:

Triscuits
Archer Farms Fruit Strips
Archer Farms Instant Oatmeal
Skippy Natural Peanut Butter
Sunsweet Plum Sweets
Clif bars
Horizon UHT Milk
Honey, Almonds, Raisins

When you get to your destination, just pick up some fresh fruit and bread. You don't have to refrigerate these items and it will save you money by not having to eat out for every meal.

Nutrition

Try Protein Shakes

If you've ever had a protein shake at a club or speciality shop, hopefully you enjoyed it. They are a great thing to drink after a workout (or anytime) because they are full of power foods, giving you a lot of bang for your buck.

Ask The Trainer

I think I eat just fine but can't lose weight. What should I do?

Keep a food diary of everything you eat. You may be surprised at how many calories you consume.

The building blocks in my shakes are whey, yogurt and ice. Whey is full of muscle repairing protein. Yogurt has several benefits, the biggest advantage being its ability to add volume and therefore helping you feel more full. Ice adds volume, water and coldness.

THE**FAT**TRAINER

Most of my shakes also include a fruit, flax seed or oatmeal, milk and peanut butter. As you add these extra ingredients to the blender, be mindful of the extra calories. They add up quickly. Try not to drink too big of a glass of these delicious power-packed treats. Also, don't be afraid to experiment with different ingredients.

Serving Size

Serving size can be difficult to figure out. It is different for everybody. I need more calories than my wife does. Measuring the food you prepare and eat is the annoying but necessary tool that will help you understand how many calories are in your servings. Don't worry though. It doesn't take too long to learn what is right for you. Your body will learn to adjust and you won't have to measure your food forever.

Nutrition

Cheating

It is useful and vital to build in one "cheat meal" per week when trying to lose weight. This cheat meal allows you to still enjoy your favorite foods even though they might not be the healthiest choice. Whatever you choose, plan for it and try to apply what you're learning about your body to your meal.

———

There are still a lot of unknowns out there regarding nutrition, but what I've found is that the closer you can get to eating whole and natural foods, the better. By controlling what you eat, you are in the driver's seat of your life. Once I got started on better nutrition, things really started to come together for me. I started losing fat pounds, shopping became easier and most importantly, my self regard improved.

THE**FAT**TRAINER

> ### *Holland's Tip*
> *To save money and avoid over eating, split an entrée with your mate.*

Nutrition

As I mentioned earlier, it took me and my wife a long time at the grocery store when we first started reading food labels and figuring out our menu.

Below is a list that we use when we go grocery shopping and as we prepare our menus for the week.

1. Oatmeal - Buy the old fashioned, plain stuff. Sweeten it with honey, fruit, etc.
2. Try to eat fish two or three times a week.
3. Milk - Fat free.
4. Try to avoid soda. If you miss it, there are some healthier bubbly drink options available.
5. Snacks - Aim for combinations of proteins with fruits, vegetables or dairy.
6. Peanut Butter - All natural.
7. Jam - Sweetened with fruit juice only.
8. Bread - 100% whole wheat/grains. You can find it without HFCS; you just have to look for it.
9. Compare the calories per slice of bread. Some slices have twice as many calories as others.
10. String Cheese - Light.
11. Try not to shop hungry.
12. Salad Dressing - Italian or olive oil and vinegar.
13. Prepare meals with olive oil or canola oil.
14. Cheese - Mozzarella is one of the best, but we mix it up, too.
15. While canned fruits and vegetables can be handy, be careful of added sugar and salt. Look for fruit canned in its own juice.

THE**FAT**TRAINER

16. If it's not in your home, you won't eat it.
17. Yogurt - All natural. We usually get low fat vanilla.
18. Flavor vegetables with olive oil, salt, pepper and spices.
19. Take your favorite recipes and alter them with healthier ingredients.
20. Popcorn - We either air pop it, or cook it in canola oil.
21. Frequently try something outside of your normal eating comfort zone. There are a lot of delicious foods out there!
22. Pasta and Couscous - 100% whole wheat.
23. Rice - Organic long grain brown.
24. Protein Shake - Watch out for portion size.
25. Salads are a great way to pack in the veggies.
26. Cereal - Look for brands without HFCS and that contain a good amount of fiber.
27. Deli Meat - Look for those marked "All Natural."
28. Drink water! Drink water! Drink water!
29. Take your kids to the grocery store. Help them learn how to be educated shoppers by having *them* select healthy foods.
30. "An apple a day..."
31. Take a multivitamin that is appropriate for your age and gender. Ask your doctor what's right for you.
32. Eating healthier may be a little more expensive, but is well worth the investment.

Nutrition

	Monday	Tuesday	Wednesday	
Breakfast	Oatmeal Raspberries Milk	Eggs Canadian Bacon Banana Milk	Cereal Raspberries Milk	
Snack	Raisins Hard Boiled Egg	Raspberry Shake	Strawberry & Banana Shake	
Lunch	Peanut Butter and Fruit Spread Sandwich String Cheese V8 Juice	Hummus Triscuits String Cheese V8 Juice	Turkey Sandwich Orange V8 Juice	
Snack	Apple Almonds	Pear Almonds	Apple String Cheese	
Dinner	Tuna Cakes w/ Flax Salad w/ Tomatoes and Avocado	Veggie Burger Sweet Potato	Angel Hair Pasta w/ Olive Oil, Feta and Fresh Tomatoes Salad w/ Cucumbers	
Snack	Yogurt Fruit Spread	Applesauce Cheese	Grapes Cheese	

THE**FAT**TRAINER

	Thursday	Friday	Saturday	Sunday
	English Muffin Fruit Spread Milk	Oatmeal Raspberries Milk	Whole Wheat Pancakes w/ Peanut Butter and Fruit Spread Milk	Cereal Banana Milk
	Yogurt Granola Raspberries	Strawberry Shake	Hummus Carrots Prunes	Applesauce Almonds
	Tuna Fish Sandwich Pear	Pizza V8 Juice Ice Cream	Blackberry Shake	Peanut Butter and Fruit Spread Sandwich String Cheese V8 Juice
	Raisins Almonds	Apple Almonds	Grapes String Cheese	Raisins Peanut Butter
	Turkey Chile w/ Flax Baked Brown Rice	Salmon Roasted Butternut Squash	Couscous Salad w/ Shrimp and Beans V8 Juice	Pork Chops w/ Blueberries Green Beans
	Apple Cheese	Cottage Cheese Pineapple	Apple Peanut Butter	Popcorn Dried Apricots

Nutrition

The meal plan on the previous page might not be practical for you. We typically eat similar meals for breakfast, lunch and snacks throughout our week. It is easier to plan that way and is less expensive. We just wanted to give you as many healthy meal ideas as possible. Below are a few more of our favorites.

Don't forget - aim to have a fruit and/or vegetable at every meal.

Breakfast

Toast with jam (fruit spread)
Omelet
Fruit salad with nuts and yogurt
Waffles (whole wheat) with peanut butter and jam
Cream of wheat
Muffins and fresh fruit

Lunch

Tomato sandwich
Tuna and avocado sandwich
Chicken roll-ups
Shrimp salad on rolls or greens
Cucumber and tomato salad
Grilled cheese
Leftovers

THE**FAT**TRAINER

Dinner

Shish kebobs
Corn chowder with whole wheat rolls
Butternut squash soup with croutons and gnocchi
Broccoli-potato soup
Quesadillas (veggie-packed)
Grilled shrimp and corn on the cob
Gyros with steak
Grilled chicken salad with grapes, almonds, mandarins
Lasagna

Snacks

Peanut butter and bananas
Cottage cheese and tomatoes
Guacamole
Almonds and raisins
Chips and salsa
Sweet potato fries (homemade)
Baked zucchini slices and mozzarella
Whey and milk
Rice pudding
Carrots and cheese
Cereal bars
Olives and mozzarella
Low-fat ice cream
Pretzels
Pine nuts
Cereal

Nutrition

Now it is your turn. Take a minute to plan out your next week of food. Having a plan made the difference for my success, and it may be for you too. Give it a try.

	Monday	Tuesday	Wednesday	
Breakfast				
Snack				
Lunch				
Snack				
Dinner				
Snack				

THE**FAT**TRAINER

Visit *TheFatTrainerBook.com/meal-plan* for a
downloadable version of this schedule.

	Thursday	Friday	Saturday	Sunday

INTANGIBLES

Winston Churchill once said, "Never, never, never give up." As most of us know, it's not always easy to live the lifestyle we know we should be living. It can get very discouraging at times when we need to kick old habits, especially if they're habits we may still enjoy. Remember that the road to a healthier lifestyle is more than just a physical one. It's very much a mental journey as well. Our minds unlock the power of our thoughts and our thoughts directly effect our actions. If we think positively about fitness, for example, we can discover the motivation we need to *be* fit. If we need to make

Intangibles

changes, we must tell ourselves that we can do it and then we must do it.

Don't get stuck on the occasional setback or failure. Take today for what it's worth and move forward. Trust me, it's easy to sleep in on a cold, wintry morning when my goal is to get up and run before work or to blow my diet on good 'ol pizza and ice-cream when I've already had my weekly allowance of it. Those things happen once in awhile, but the important thing is that I recommit in my mind to stick to my goals and then follow through.

Holland's Tip
Learning how to live healthy takes time so be patient with yourself. Changing old habits will not happen overnight.

Prayer and meditation are two other very important components of this mental journey that I use alongside my fitness routine. By taking the time to commune with my inner-self and with my Creator, my mind and soul are given the chance to be revived and I regain focus on my goals.

> **"A man is but the product of his thoughts. What he thinks, he becomes."**
>
> *-Gandhi*

Prayer and meditation are also vital in helping us be relaxed. We all have our own ways to relax (like reading a book or watching TV), but try the following some time. Go to a quiet and private place. Sit in a comfortable position. Close your eyes. Breathe slowly and just 'chill.' If you're not into praying or meditating, this might feel awkward, but I guarantee that you will find positive results. Reflect on all the blessings you have such as a body that works, your senses, your family, your freedom, your shelter and food, etc. Verbally ask for help from your Creator to help you with your fitness goals and whatever other goals you may have. As we learn how to better relax both our minds and our bodies, we will

Intangibles

see very distinct improvements in our lifestyles. Constant prayer and meditation in my day-to-day routine makes a huge difference!

A deeper and more intense form of prayer and meditation is fasting. On the first Sunday of every month, I complete a twenty-four-hour fast. I refrain from eating food or drinking liquid (including water) for one day and I do *not* exercise. I use this time to complete my normal routine and rededicate myself to my personal goals that month (whether they are fitness related or not). Every time I feel hungry, I take a moment to think about my goals and determine how I can better reach them. I begin and end each fast with prayer.

Ask The Trainer

How do I stay motivated?

Find someone who will support you in your new behaviors. Choose someone who can both sympathize with you and encourage you.

THE**FAT**TRAINER

Whether or not you feel comfortable with these suggestions, remember to take time out of each day to relax and rejuvenate. Be positive in your thoughts and keep moving forward with your goals. These "intangibles" have the potential of changing your life!

G O A L S

I am certainly not the first person to say this, but I'll say it anyway. Set goals! Among other reasons for setting goals, it's important to know why you're doing what you're trying to do. You need to have an end in mind. Setting goals helps you see progress and improvement in yourself. It's also something to fall back on when you need a little extra motivation.

For me, setting and achieving goals has turned a lifetime challenge of being overweight into a newfound strength. For my fitness needs, I still set long term and short term goals. My fitness journey is not yet over, nor will it ever really be. My long term goals include a total scale weight loss, body fat loss, clothes size and mile time. My short term goals

Goals

include things like one to two pounds of weight loss per week, getting up before work to run and only eating ice cream once per week.

Getting with a trainer can help you determine how to achieve your particular goals. Remember that while scale weight is a fine goal to go by, body fat is ultimately the better standard to use. If possible, try to measure your body fat every four to eight weeks.

Ask The Trainer

How do you get over the initial drag of getting back into shape?

Here are a couple of ideas:
Hire a trainer.
Start light and brief.
Do what you enjoy most.
e.g. Play ball, dance, swim.

This will give you a much better guide to see how you are doing, even if you're not trying to lose weight.

For goals that pertain to weight loss and losing inches, it is acceptable to weigh or measure yourself every week or two. My wife uses a measuring tape to track inches lost around my neck, shoulders, chest, abs, waist, arms and legs. When I don't see a scale weight change, this form of measurement really helps me stay motivated because I can see the inches lost. Again, try to refrain from stepping on that scale more than one time per week. It can be discouraging because weight can naturally fluctuate from day to day.

"Obstacles are those frightening things that become visible when we take our eyes off our goals."

-Henry Ford

Rewards

The rewards you receive from achieving your goals are just as important as the goals themselves. The great thing about rewards is that you choose them. Just as a child is positively rewarded for the good thing he or she does, an adult can benefit from

Goals

this reinforcement, too. It's ideal for the reward to match the activity that achieved it. So things like clothes, treats, toys or a night out may be a good fit for fat loss. Just be careful not to over or under reward yourself. A good pat on the back may be just the thing for losing a pound in a week; whereas a family trip to the beach may be just the thing when you lose 15 percent body fat.

THE **FAT** TRAINER

THE FAT TRAINER

"One day a hare saw a tortoise walking slowly along and began to laugh and mock him. The hare challenged the tortoise to a race and the tortoise accepted. They agreed on a route and started the race. The hare shot ahead and ran briskly for some time. Then seeing that he was far ahead of the tortoise, he thought he'd sit under a tree for some time and relax before continuing the race.

He sat under the tree and soon fell asleep. The tortoise, plodding on, overtook him and finished the race. The hare woke up and realized that he had lost the race.

Holland Newton

The moral... 'Slow and steady wins the race.'"

This fable, as taken from Wikipedia, illustrates the years it took to change my habits and mind-set in regards to health and fitness. I took each change one step at a time and was persistent, just like the tortoise. The changes I made over time weren't easy and I'm not perfect, but my family and I are on track to living a life of fullness, health, fitness and wellness.

As you implement these new or modified behaviors into your life, you'll find not only improved physical health, but your entire life will improve and you'll be happier for it.

Good luck and God bless,

Holland - The (not as) Fat Trainer

THE **FAT** TRAINER

Notes & Thoughts

THE **FAT** TRAINER

Notes & Thoughts

THE**FAT**TRAINER

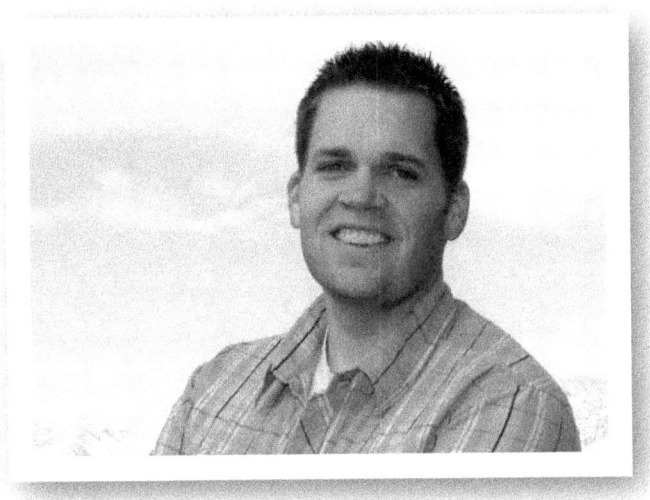

Holland was born in September 1981 in Salt Lake City and raised in Columbia, Missouri. He holds a Bachelors of Journalism and Master of Arts from the University of Missouri.

While studying advertising at Mizzou, he worked at Wilson's Fitness Centers as a personal trainer. He is certified with NESTA (National Exercise & Sports Trainers Association). He played college football and lacrosse, lived in England and loves being outdoors.

When he's not writing awesome fitness books, Holland is a communications strategist in the branding and marketing field.

Holland currently lives in Salt Lake City with his wife, Jennifer and son, Ethan.